JUMPING EXERCISE

FOR BEGINNERS

The Ultimate Guide To Effective Workouts, Improving Cardiovascular Health, Building Strength, And Enhancing Agility With Simple, Easy-To-Follow Routines

ROBERT LUGO

CHAPTER 1
Introduction To Jumping Exercises

Jumping exercises are a foundational aspect of many fitness routines, whether you're a beginner or a seasoned athlete. They encompass a wide range of movements, from simple jumps like jumping jacks to more complex plyometric exercises. These exercises are not only fun but also highly effective in improving cardiovascular fitness, muscle strength, and overall athleticism. In this discussion, we'll delve into the concepts of jumping exercises for beginners, exploring the benefits, safety considerations, precautions, and equipment needed to perform these exercises effectively.

Understanding the Benefits of Jumping

Jumping exercises offer a plethora of benefits that contribute to overall health and fitness. One of the primary advantages is their cardiovascular impact. When you engage in jumping exercises, your heart rate increases, promoting better cardiovascular endurance over time. This improved cardiovascular health not only benefits your workouts but also enhances your daily activities, making tasks like climbing stairs or carrying groceries easier.

Moreover, jumping exercises are excellent for burning calories and aiding in weight management. The dynamic nature of these exercises engages multiple muscle groups simultaneously, leading to a higher calorie burn compared to static exercises. This calorie expenditure can contribute significantly to weight loss or weight maintenance goals when combined with a balanced diet.

Another significant benefit of jumping exercises is their impact on lower body strength and power. These exercises target muscles such as the quadriceps, hamstrings, calves, and glutes, leading to improved muscle tone, strength, and endurance.

As a beginner, focusing on foundational jumping exercises can help you build a strong lower body foundation, which is essential for various sports and daily activities.

Additionally, jumping exercises enhance proprioception and balance. Proprioception refers to your body's ability to sense its position and movement in space. By incorporating jumps into your routine, you challenge your proprioceptive abilities, leading to improved balance and coordination. This aspect is particularly beneficial for older adults looking to maintain functional independence and reduce the risk of falls.

Furthermore, jumping exercises can have a positive impact on bone health. Weight-bearing activities like jumping stimulate bone remodeling, leading to increased bone density and strength. This is especially crucial for individuals at risk of osteoporosis or those looking to prevent age-related bone loss.

In summary, the benefits of jumping exercises for beginners are multifaceted. They improve cardiovascular fitness, aid in weight management, strengthen lower body muscles, enhance balance and coordination, and promote bone health. Incorporating these exercises into your routine can have a transformative effect on your overall health and fitness levels.

Safety Considerations and Precautions

While jumping exercises offer numerous benefits, it's essential to approach them with caution, especially as a beginner. Safety considerations and precautions play a crucial role in preventing injuries and ensuring a positive exercise experience.

First and foremost, it's essential to start slowly and gradually increase the intensity of your jumping exercises. Jumping places significant stress on your joints and muscles, so rushing into high-impact jumps without proper conditioning can lead to injuries such as sprains, strains, or stress fractures.

Begin with low-impact jumps like jumping jacks or gentle hops, and progressively add more challenging variations as your strength and fitness improve.

Proper technique is paramount when performing jumping exercises. Focus on maintaining good form throughout each jump to minimize the risk of injury. For instance, when performing squat jumps, ensure that your knees track in line with your toes and that you land softly with bent knees to absorb the impact.

It's also crucial to listen to your body and avoid pushing through pain or discomfort. If you experience sharp pain, especially in your joints, stop the exercise immediately and consult a healthcare professional if needed. Ignoring pain signals can exacerbate injuries and prolong recovery time.

Furthermore, consider the surface on which you perform jumping exercises. Opt for a flat, cushioned surface to reduce impact on your joints. Avoid concrete or other hard surfaces, as they can increase the risk of injuries like shin splints or joint pain.

Warm-up and cool-down are essential components of any exercise routine, including jumping exercises. Begin with a dynamic warm-up to prepare your muscles and joints for the demands of jumping. This can include activities like jogging in place, leg swings, and arm circles. After your workout, engage in a thorough cool-down consisting of stretching exercises to promote flexibility and reduce muscle soreness.

Incorporating variety into your jumping exercises can also help prevent overuse injuries. Alternate between different types of jumps, such as vertical jumps, lateral jumps, and box jumps, to distribute the workload across various muscle groups and reduce strain on specific areas.

Lastly, see a physician if you have any past injuries or medical issues.

Healthcare professional or a certified fitness trainer before starting a jumping exercise program. They can provide personalized guidance and modifications to ensure a safe and effective workout regimen.

By following these safety considerations and precautions, you can enjoy the benefits of jumping exercises while minimizing the risk of injuries, making your fitness journey both rewarding and sustainable.

Equipment Needed for Jumping Exercises

Jumping exercises can be performed with minimal equipment, making them accessible to beginners and seasoned fitness enthusiasts alike. However, certain pieces of equipment can enhance your jumping workout experience and provide additional options for variation and progression.

One of the most basic pieces of equipment for jumping exercises is athletic footwear. Invest in a pair of well-fitted athletic shoes with good cushioning and support, especially if you plan to perform high-impact jumps. Proper footwear can reduce the risk of foot and ankle injuries and improve your overall comfort during workouts.

A jump rope is another versatile and affordable piece of equipment for jumping exercises. Jump ropes offer an excellent cardiovascular workout and can be used to perform various jump rope exercises, such as single jumps, double unders, and criss-cross jumps. They are portable and can be used indoors or outdoors, making them a convenient option for home workouts or on-the-go fitness routines.

For more advanced jumping exercises, consider incorporating plyometric boxes or platforms. These sturdy boxes come in different heights and can be used for exercises like box jumps, step-ups, and depth jumps.

Plyometric boxes provide a challenging way to improve lower body strength, power, and explosiveness.

Resistance bands are another valuable addition to your jumping exercise equipment arsenal.

These elastic bands come in different resistance levels and can be used to add resistance to jumping exercises, such as lateral band walks, squat jumps with bands, and resisted high knees.

Resistance bands are lightweight, portable, and suitable for targeting specific muscle groups during jumps.

If you have access to a gym or fitness facility, consider using foam mats or padded flooring for jumping exercises. These surfaces offer cushioning and shock absorption, reducing the impact on your joints during high-impact jumps.

They are especially beneficial for individuals with joint issues or those recovering from injuries.

Incorporating a stability ball into your jumping workout can also add variety and challenge. Stability balls can be used for exercises like stability ball squats, ball slams, and plank jumps.

They engage your core muscles and improve balance and stability, enhancing the overall effectiveness of your jumping exercises.

Additionally, consider using a timer or stopwatch to track your rest intervals and workout duration during jumping exercises. Structuring your workouts with timed intervals can help maintain intensity and motivation, leading to better results over time.

While these equipment options can enhance your jumping exercise routine, remember that you can still achieve a great workout with just your body weight.

Focus on mastering proper form and technique before incorporating additional equipment or increasing intensity.

As you progress, gradually introduce new equipment and variations to keep your workouts challenging and engaging.

CHAPTER 2
Anatomy And Physiology Of Jumping

Jumping exercises for beginners involve a complex interplay of anatomy and physiology to generate the power and coordination needed for effective jumps.

Understanding the underlying mechanisms can greatly enhance performance and reduce the risk of injury. Let's delve into the anatomy and physiology of jumping, including the muscles involved, joint mechanics, range of motion, and energy systems at play.

Muscles Involved in Jumping Movements:

Jumping requires the coordinated effort of various muscle groups to generate propulsion, stabilize the body, and control landing. The primary muscles involved can be categorized into three main groups:

1. Lower Body Muscles:

o Quadriceps: The quadriceps, including the rectus femoris, vastus lateralis, vastus medialis, and vastus intermedius, play a crucial role in extending the knee during the upward phase of the jump.

o Hamstrings: The hamstrings, comprising the biceps femoris, semitendinosus, and semimembranosus, assist in hip extension and knee flexion during the push-off phase.

o Gluteal Muscles: The gluteus maximus, medius, and minimus contribute to hip extension and provide stability during takeoff and landing.

o Calves: The gastrocnemius and soleus muscles are essential for plantar flexion of the ankle, aiding in pushing off the ground and achieving height in the jump.

2. Core Muscles:

o Abdominals: The rectus abdominis, obliques, and transverse abdominis help stabilize the torso and transfer force from the lower body to the upper body during jumping.

o Lower Back: The erector spinae muscles provide spinal support and assist in maintaining an upright posture throughout the jump.

3. Upper Body Muscles:

o Deltoids and Pectorals: These muscles contribute to arm swing and balance during the jump, especially in exercises like the vertical jump where arm movement plays a significant role.

o Trapezius and Rhomboids: These muscles help stabilize the shoulders and upper back, enhancing overall posture and control during jumping movements.

Joint Mechanics and Range of Motion:

Jumping involves dynamic movements at multiple joints, each with its specific range of motion and function:

1. Ankle Joint:

o Dorsiflexion: During the pre-loading phase of the jump, dorsiflexion (lifting the toes towards the shin) allows for optimal foot positioning and energy storage in the calf muscles.

o Plantar Flexion: The explosive push-off phase is facilitated by plantar flexion (pointing the toes downward), activating the calf muscles and propelling the body upward.

2. Knee Joint:

o Flexion and Extension: The knee flexes during the downward phase of the jump, storing elastic energy in the quadriceps and hamstrings. Extension occurs rapidly during takeoff, generating upward thrust.

3. Hip Joint:

o Flexion and Extension: Hip flexion occurs as the body descends into the jump, while hip extension drives the upward movement, powered by the gluteal and hamstring muscles.

4. Spine and Pelvis:

o Neutral Spine: Maintaining a neutral spine position is crucial for distributing forces evenly and minimizing stress on the lower back.

o Pelvic Stability: Proper engagement of core muscles ensures pelvic stability, optimizing power transfer from the lower body to the upper body.

Energy Systems Used in Jumping:

Jumping exercises primarily rely on the anaerobic energy systems, specifically the ATP-PCr system and the glycolytic system, due to the explosive nature and short duration of jumps.

1. ATP-PCr System:

o Immediate Energy: The ATP-PCr system provides rapid energy through the breakdown of phosphocreatine (PCr) to replenish adenosine triphosphate (ATP) stores.

o High-Intensity Output: This system fuels quick, high-intensity movements like the initial burst of force in a jump, lasting for several seconds before fatigue sets in.

2. Glycolytic System:

o Short-Term Energy: As the ATP-PCr system diminishes, the glycolytic system kicks in, breaking down glucose for ATP production through anaerobic glycolysis.

o Lactic Acid Accumulation: Intense jumping activities can lead to lactic acid accumulation, causing fatigue and muscle burn after repeated efforts or sustained high-intensity jumps.

CHAPTER 3
Principles Of Effective Jump Training

Jump training for beginners is founded on several key principles that are essential for safe and productive workouts. These principles encompass progressive overload and adaptation, proper form and technique, as well as the crucial aspect of recovery and rest.

Progressive Overload and Adaptation

One of the foundational principles of effective jump training is the concept of progressive overload. This principle revolves around gradually increasing the intensity, duration, or frequency of your jumping exercises over time. By challenging your muscles and cardiovascular system progressively, you stimulate growth and improvement. This gradual progression allows your body to adapt to increasing demands, leading to gains in strength, power, and endurance.

Implementing progressive overload in jump training involves various strategies.

You can increase the height or distance of your jumps, add resistance through weights or resistance bands, or modify the complexity of the jumping movements.

It's crucial to find the right balance between challenge and safety, ensuring that you push yourself without risking injury.

Adaptation is closely tied to progressive overload. As you consistently expose your body to increased demands through jumping exercises, it adapts by becoming stronger, more resilient, and better coordinated.

These adaptations occur at the muscular, skeletal, and neuromuscular levels, enhancing your overall athletic performance and functional abilities.

Proper Form and Technique

Proper form and technique are paramount in jump training, especially for beginners. Correct form not only maximizes the effectiveness of your workouts but also reduces the risk of injuries. When performing jumping exercises, focus on:

1. Alignment: Maintain proper alignment of your body throughout each jump. Keep your knees in line with your toes, engage your core muscles, and avoid excessive arching or rounding of your back.

2. Landing Mechanics: Pay attention to how you land after each jump. Land softly with bent knees to absorb shock, distribute the impact evenly across your feet, and avoid landing with locked joints.

3. Arm Movement: Coordinate your arm movements with your jumps. Swing your arms naturally to generate momentum and assist in

propulsion, but avoid excessive swinging that can disrupt your balance.

4. Breathing: Practice rhythmic breathing during jumps. Inhale before the jump, exhale during the effort phase (e.g., when pushing off the ground), and continue to breathe steadily throughout the movement.

Consistent practice and mindful attention to proper form and technique not only enhance the effectiveness of your jump training but also reduce the risk of overuse injuries or strain on joints and muscles.

Recovery and Rest for Jump Training

While the intensity of jump training is beneficial for stimulating progress, adequate recovery and rest are equally essential for optimal results. Recovery encompasses various aspects that promote healing, repair, and adaptation following intense workouts. Key elements of recovery for jump training include:

1. Sleep: Quality sleep is crucial for recovery and overall well-being. Aim for 7-9 hours of uninterrupted sleep per night to support muscle repair, hormone regulation, and cognitive function.

2. Nutrition: Fuel your body with a balanced diet rich in protein, complex carbohydrates, healthy fats, vitamins, and minerals. Adequate nutrition supports muscle recovery, replenishes glycogen stores, and boosts energy levels for training sessions.

3. Active Recovery: Incorporate light activities such as walking, stretching, or low-impact exercises on rest days. Active recovery promotes blood flow, reduces muscle stiffness, and aids in recovery without causing additional fatigue.

4. Recovery Techniques: Explore various recovery techniques such as foam rolling, massage, contrast baths, or using compression garments. These methods can help alleviate muscle

soreness, improve circulation, and enhance recovery between training sessions.

5. Listen to Your Body: Pay attention to signs of fatigue, soreness, or overtraining. Adjust your training intensity, volume, or frequency as needed to prevent burnout and allow sufficient recovery time.

By prioritizing recovery and rest alongside your jump training regimen, you support your body's ability to adapt, grow stronger, and perform at its best over time. Incorporate these principles systematically into your workouts to maximize the benefits of jump training while minimizing the risk of injuries or setbacks.

CHAPTER 4
Types Of Jumping Exercises

Vertical jumps are fundamental in developing lower body strength, explosiveness, and vertical leap height. Techniques such as the squat jump, tuck jump, and split squat jump are effective for beginners. The squat jump involves bending the knees and hips, then explosively extending them to jump vertically. Tuck jumps add a dynamic element by bringing the knees to the chest mid-air. Split squat jumps focus on unilateral leg strength, aiding in balance and coordination development.

Horizontal jumps focus on horizontal displacement and lower body power. Techniques like the broad jump, lateral jumps, and bounding variations enhance agility and speed. The broad jump involves a powerful push-off to propel forward, emphasizing hip and leg coordination. Lateral jumps improve lateral quickness and stability, crucial for sports like basketball or soccer.

Bounding exercises combine vertical and horizontal elements, challenging leg muscles in multiple planes of motion.

Plyometric drills are integral for building explosive power through rapid muscle contraction. Exercises like depth jumps, box jumps, and jump squats improve fast-twitch muscle fibers' recruitment and neuromuscular coordination. Depth jumps involve stepping off a box, landing softly, and then immediately jumping vertically. Box jumps require jumping onto a platform, enhancing vertical leaps and landing mechanics. Jump squats combine squatting with explosive jumps, targeting lower body strength and power development.

Understanding these types of jumping exercises allows beginners to structure their workouts effectively, progressing from basic to more advanced variations. Incorporating proper technique, progression, and recovery ensures optimal gains in strength, power, and athletic performance.

CHAPTER 5
Designing Jumping Workouts

Designing effective jumping workouts for beginners involves a systematic approach that considers various factors such as fitness level, goals, safety, and progression.

A well-designed jumping workout not only enhances cardiovascular fitness but also improves muscular strength, power, and coordination.

The first step in designing jumping workouts is to assess the individual's current fitness level and any specific goals they may have.

Beginners should start with basic jumps like two-footed jumps, focusing on proper technique and landing mechanics to prevent injuries.

As they progress, more advanced jumps such as single-leg jumps or box jumps can be introduced gradually.

Structuring Jump Training Sessions

Structuring jump training sessions involves organizing exercises, sets, reps, and rest periods to optimize performance and minimize fatigue and injury risk. A typical jump training session may include a warm-up, main workout segment, and cool-down.

Warm-up: The warm-up phase should include dynamic stretches, light cardio exercises, and mobility drills to prepare the muscles, joints, and nervous system for the upcoming workout.

Main Workout: The main workout segment comprises a variety of jumping exercises targeting different muscle groups and movement patterns. It's essential to include a mix of vertical jumps, lateral jumps, and plyometric exercises to develop overall explosiveness and agility.

Cool-down: The cool-down phase involves stretching exercises, foam rolling, and relaxation techniques to promote recovery, reduce muscle soreness, and improve flexibility.

Incorporating Jumping into Full-Body Workouts

Integrating jumping exercises into full-body workouts offers a holistic approach to fitness by engaging multiple muscle groups simultaneously. This not only improves overall strength and endurance but also enhances coordination and balance.

A well-rounded full-body workout incorporating jumping exercises may include:

1. Lower Body Focus: Incorporate exercises like squat jumps, lunge jumps, and box jumps to target the lower body muscles including quadriceps, hamstrings, glutes, and calves.

2. Upper Body Engagement: Combine jumping exercises with upper body movements such as burpees with a push-up or medicine ball slams to engage the arms, chest, shoulders, and core.

3. Core Stability: Include exercises like plank jumps or mountain climbers to challenge core stability and improve overall functional strength.

4. Circuit Training: Design circuit-style workouts alternating between jumping exercises and strength or cardio exercises to maximize calorie burn and improve cardiovascular fitness.

Progression Strategies for Beginners

Progression is key in jump training to ensure continuous improvement and prevent plateaus or overtraining. Beginners should start with low-impact jumps and gradually increase intensity, volume, and complexity over time.

Some progression strategies for beginners include:

1. Gradual Intensity Increase: Begin with basic jumps and gradually increase intensity by adding height, distance, or resistance (e.g., using weighted vests or ankle weights).

2. Incremental Volume: Start with a manageable number of sets and reps and gradually increase as strength and endurance improve. However, avoid excessive volume to prevent overuse injuries.

3. Technique Mastery: Emphasize proper technique and landing mechanics before progressing to more challenging jumps. Focus on quality over quantity to ensure safety and effectiveness.

4. Rest and Recovery: Allow adequate rest between jump training sessions to promote recovery and prevent fatigue-related injuries. Incorporate active recovery activities like swimming or yoga on rest days.

By implementing these progression strategies and designing well-structured jump workouts, beginners can safely and effectively improve their jumping abilities, overall fitness, and athletic performance over time.

CHAPTER 6
Combining Jumping With Other Exercises

Integrating Jumping with Strength Training:

Integrating jumping exercises with strength training can create a dynamic and effective workout regimen for beginners. By combining these two modalities, individuals can enhance their overall fitness level, improve muscle strength, power, and explosiveness, and boost their cardiovascular endurance. One of the key benefits of integrating jumping with strength training is the ability to engage multiple muscle groups simultaneously, leading to efficient and comprehensive workouts.

When integrating jumping with strength training, it's essential to consider the principles of progressive overload and proper technique.

Beginners should start with basic jumping exercises like squat jumps, box jumps, and split jumps, gradually increasing intensity and complexity as they build strength and coordination. Incorporating variations such as single-leg jumps, depth jumps and lateral jumps can further challenge balance, stability, and agility while targeting different muscle groups.

Incorporating resistance into jumping exercises can also enhance strength development. Utilizing resistance bands, weighted vests, or holding dumbbells during jump squats adds external load, increasing the demand on muscles and promoting greater strength gains. Additionally, performing plyometric exercises like depth jumps or bounding drills can improve the stretch-shortening cycle, enhancing muscular power and explosiveness.

Proper form and technique are crucial when combining jumping with strength training to prevent injuries and optimize results.

Beginners should focus on landing softly with knees bent to absorb impact, maintaining a neutral spine, and engaging core muscles throughout each jump. Gradually increasing jump height, distance, or speed can further challenge the body and stimulate continuous improvement.

Overall, integrating jumping exercises with strength training offers a holistic approach to fitness, targeting various aspects of physical performance and promoting functional strength and athleticism for beginners.

Adding Cardiovascular Elements to Jump Workouts:

Incorporating cardiovascular elements into jump workouts not only enhances aerobic fitness but also adds variety and intensity to training sessions. By combining jumping exercises with cardio intervals, beginners can improve cardiovascular endurance, burn calories, and boost overall stamina.

To add cardiovascular elements to jump workouts, incorporating high-intensity interval training (HIIT) can be highly effective. Alternating between periods of intense jumping exercises and active recovery, such as jogging in place or jumping rope, creates a challenging yet manageable workout structure. This approach not only elevates heart rate and increases calorie expenditure but also enhances the metabolic response, leading to improved cardiovascular health and fat burning.

Incorporating plyometric drills like jump squats, burpees, or ladder drills with short rest intervals between sets can create an intense cardiovascular workout while targeting muscular endurance and power. Beginners should focus on maintaining proper form and breathing rhythm throughout each exercise to optimize cardiovascular benefits and minimize fatigue.

Additionally, integrating jump rope exercises into jump workouts can further enhance cardiovascular conditioning.

Jumping rope engages multiple muscle groups, improves coordination and agility, and boosts heart rate, making it an excellent complement to jumping exercises. Beginners can start with basic jump rope techniques and progress to more advanced variations like double unders or alternating foot jumps for increased intensity.

Proper warm-up and cool-down periods are essential when adding cardiovascular elements to jump workouts to prevent injury and facilitate recovery. Incorporating dynamic stretches, mobility exercises, and foam rolling can help prepare the body for intense activity and promote muscle relaxation post-workout.

Overall, adding cardiovascular elements to jump workouts offers a comprehensive approach to fitness, combining strength, power, agility, and endurance for beginners seeking versatile and effective training routines.

Functional Movement Patterns and Jumping:

Understanding functional movement patterns and their relationship to jumping exercises is essential for beginners to develop balanced and efficient movement patterns, improve athletic performance, and reduce the risk of injury. Functional movements involve multiple joints and muscles working together to perform tasks commonly encountered in daily activities or sports.

When incorporating functional movement patterns into jumping exercises, it's important to focus on movements that mimic real-life activities and promote optimal biomechanics. Squatting, lunging, pushing, pulling, twisting, and bending are fundamental functional movements that can be integrated into jump workouts to enhance overall movement quality and functionality.

For example, combining squatting movements like jump squats or squat jumps with upper-body pushing exercises such as medicine ball throws or plyometric push-ups engages both lower and upper body muscles, promoting full-body coordination and strength development. Similarly, incorporating jumping lunges or split jumps with rotational movements like medicine ball twists or woodchoppers challenges core stability, balance, and agility while improving functional movement patterns.

Functional movement-based circuits can be an effective way for beginners to integrate functional movements with jumping exercises.

Designing circuits that include a variety of movements targeting different planes of motion and muscle groups ensures a comprehensive and balanced workout. Incorporating equipment such as stability balls, resistance bands, or TRX straps can add variability and challenge to functional jump training.

Moreover, focusing on proper movement mechanics and alignment during functional jump exercises is crucial for injury prevention and optimal performance. Beginners should emphasize maintaining a neutral spine, proper knee alignment, and engaging core muscles to ensure the safe and effective execution of movements.

By incorporating functional movement patterns into jumping exercises, beginners can enhance overall movement proficiency, athleticism, and functional strength, leading to improved performance in daily activities, sports, and fitness pursuits.

CHAPTER 7
Common Mistakes And How To Avoid Them

In jumping exercises for beginners, avoiding common mistakes is crucial for progress, safety, and long-term success. One of the primary concerns is overtraining and injury prevention. Beginners may be enthusiastic and eager to see rapid results, leading them to push too hard or train too frequently without allowing sufficient rest and recovery time. This can result in overuse injuries like shin splints, tendonitis, or stress fractures. To avoid this, it's essential to emphasize the importance of gradual progression, rest days, and listening to one's body for signs of fatigue or strain.

Another significant aspect of avoiding mistakes in jumping exercises is correcting form errors. Poor form not only reduces the effectiveness of the exercise but also increases the risk of injury.

Beginners may struggle with proper landing techniques, such as landing with stiff knees or letting the knees collapse inward, which can strain the joints and lead to injuries like ACL tears or patellar tendinitis. By focusing on teaching correct form from the start, emphasizing the importance of soft landings, proper knee alignment, and using the whole foot to absorb impact, beginners can reduce the risk of injury and optimize their performance.

Monitoring progress and adjusting intensity is another key concept in avoiding common mistakes in jumping exercises. Beginners often fall into the trap of sticking to the same routine without tracking their progress or adjusting the intensity of their workouts. This can lead to plateaus in performance and prevent them from reaching their full potential. Encouraging beginners to keep a workout journal, track their repetitions, sets, and rest periods, and gradually increase the intensity or difficulty of their exercises over time can help them avoid stagnation and continue making progress safely.

Overall, in jumping exercises for beginners, a focus on preventing overtraining and injuries, correcting form errors, monitoring progress, and adjusting intensity is essential for a successful and sustainable training program. By emphasizing these concepts and providing guidance and support, beginners can build a strong foundation, improve their skills, and enjoy the benefits of jumping exercises while minimizing the risk of setbacks or injuries.

CHAPTER 8
Nutrition And Hydration For Jump Training

Fueling the body for optimal performance in jump training involves a strategic approach to nutrition that supports energy production, muscle function, and recovery. Carbohydrates are a key component, providing the primary source of fuel for intense physical activity like jumping exercises.

Complex carbohydrates such as whole grains, fruits, and vegetables offer sustained energy release, while simple carbohydrates like fruits can provide quick energy before a workout. Balancing carbohydrates with proteins is important for muscle repair and growth. Lean proteins like chicken, fish, tofu, and legumes support muscle recovery and help maintain muscle mass during training.

Hydration strategies are crucial for jump workouts, as dehydration can impair performance and increase the risk of injuries.

Water is necessary for lubricating joints, controlling body temperature, and delivering nutrients to cells. Before a jump training session, it's important to hydrate adequately by drinking water throughout the day and consuming fluids with electrolytes if exercising in hot or humid conditions.

During the workout, sipping water regularly helps maintain hydration levels. Electrolyte drinks can be beneficial for longer or more intense sessions to replenish electrolytes lost through sweat.

Post-workout nutrition plays a vital role in recovery after jump training. Consuming a combination of carbohydrates and proteins within the first 30 minutes to an hour after a workout helps replenish glycogen stores and supports muscle repair. A post-workout meal or snack could include a mix of carbohydrates like whole grains or fruits and proteins like lean meats, eggs, or protein shakes. Including foods rich in antioxidants and anti-inflammatory nutrients can also aid in reducing muscle soreness and promoting recovery. Hydrating adequately post-workout is equally important to replace fluids lost during exercise and support overall recovery processes.

CHAPTER 9
Mental Strategies For Jump Training

Mental strategies play a crucial role in jump training, especially for beginners looking to improve their performance and skills.

Here, we delve into three key concepts that can significantly enhance the effectiveness of jump training: focus and concentration techniques, visualization and mental rehearsal, and building confidence and mental toughness.

Focus and Concentration Techniques: Effective jump training requires a high level of focus and concentration to execute movements accurately and efficiently. One technique to enhance focus is mindfulness meditation. This practice involves being fully present in the moment, clearing the mind of distractions, and directing full attention to the task at hand—jumping. By incorporating mindfulness into jump training sessions, beginners can improve their ability to stay focused, leading to better technique and performance.

Another useful technique is the use of cues and reminders. These can be visual or auditory cues that prompt the athlete to maintain proper form, execute jumps with precision, and stay mentally engaged throughout the training session. For example, a visual cue could be a specific marker or line on the ground that reminds the jumper to land with correct alignment and posture.

Visualization and Mental Rehearsal: Visualization and mental rehearsal are powerful tools in jump training that involve creating vivid mental images of successful jumps and performances.

Athletes can visualize themselves executing flawless jumps, feeling the movements, sensations, and emotions associated with a successful jump. This mental practice helps reinforce neural pathways related to jump movements, leading to improved muscle memory and performance.

Mental rehearsal goes beyond visualization by incorporating detailed mental simulations of jump sequences, focusing on timing, rhythm, and coordination. By mentally rehearsing jump routines, beginners can develop a deeper understanding of the movements and improve their ability to execute them effectively when performing physically.

Building Confidence and Mental Toughness: Confidence plays a vital role in jump training, influencing motivation, persistence, and performance outcomes. Beginners can build confidence through incremental progress and achievement. Setting achievable goals and celebrating small victories can boost confidence and motivation, encouraging continued effort and improvement in jump training.

Additionally, developing mental toughness is essential for overcoming challenges and setbacks in jump training. Mental toughness involves resilience, perseverance, and the ability to maintain focus and determination despite difficulties. Techniques such as positive self-talk, reframing challenges as opportunities for growth, and maintaining a strong belief in one's abilities can help build mental toughness in jump training.

mental strategies are integral to the success of jump training for beginners.

By incorporating focus and concentration techniques, visualization and mental rehearsal, and building confidence and mental toughness, beginners can enhance their performance, improve skill acquisition, and achieve their jump training goals effectively.

CHAPTER 10
Long-Term Success In Jump Training

Setting Realistic Goals and Tracking
Progress

One of the fundamental pillars of long-term
success in jump training is the establishment of
realistic goals and the diligent tracking
of progress. Setting realistic goals involves
understanding one's current level of fitness,
considering individual capabilities and
limitations, and defining clear, achievable
objectives.

This process requires a balance between ambition
and practicality to ensure that goals are
challenging yet attainable.

When setting goals for jump training, it's essential
to consider various factors such as the specific
types of jumps being trained (e.g., vertical jumps,
broad jumps, plyometric exercises), the frequency

and intensity of training sessions, and the desired outcomes (e.g., increased vertical leap, improved explosive power, enhanced overall athleticism). Goals can be categorized into short-term, medium-term, and long-term objectives, each contributing to the overarching goal of continuous improvement.

Tracking progress plays a crucial role in maintaining motivation and gauging the effectiveness of training efforts. This involves regularly assessing key performance metrics such as jump height, distance, speed, and overall agility. Utilizing tools like jump measurement devices, video analysis, and training logs can provide quantitative data to evaluate progress objectively.

Handling Stagnation and Obstacles

In the journey towards long-term success in jump training, encountering plateaus and setbacks is not uncommon. Plateaus refer to periods where progress seems to stall or slow down despite consistent training efforts. Setbacks, on the other hand, may arise from injuries, overtraining, or external factors that disrupt the training routine. Effectively managing plateaus and setbacks is essential to maintaining momentum and staying on track with long-term goals.

To overcome plateaus, it's crucial to incorporate variety and progression into the training regimen. This can include introducing new exercises, adjusting intensity levels, incorporating periodization techniques, and focusing on weaknesses or areas that need improvement. Cross-training and incorporating complementary exercises can also prevent stagnation and keep workouts engaging and effective.

When facing setbacks such as injuries or temporary disruptions to training, it's vital to prioritize recovery and rehabilitation. This may involve consulting with healthcare professionals, modifying the training program to accommodate recovery needs, and practicing patience and resilience during the healing process.

Maintaining a positive mindset and focusing on long-term progress rather than short-term setbacks is key to overcoming challenges and staying committed to the journey.

Maintaining Motivation and Discipline

Sustaining motivation and discipline are essential components of long-term success in jump training. Motivation fuels enthusiasm, determination, and perseverance, while discipline ensures consistency, adherence to training schedules, and the ability to push through obstacles.

To maintain motivation, it's beneficial to have clear reasons and intrinsic motivations for engaging in jump training. This could include personal goals such as improving athletic performance, enhancing overall fitness, or achieving specific milestones. Setting rewards for reaching milestones can also provide incentives and reinforce positive behaviors.

Developing discipline involves establishing a structured training routine, prioritizing workouts, and cultivating habits that support long-term success. This includes setting aside dedicated time for training, creating a conducive environment for exercise, managing distractions, and staying accountable to oneself or a support system.

Incorporating motivational strategies such as visualization, positive self-talk, and goal reminders can help reinforce motivation during challenging times. Additionally, seeking support from coaches, training partners, or online communities can provide encouragement, accountability, and a sense of camaraderie in the pursuit of long-term success in jump training.

CHAPTER 11

Case Studies And Success Stories

Case studies and success stories in the realm of jumping exercises for beginners offer profound insights into the transformative power of disciplined training and determination.

Through these narratives, we witness the journey of individuals who have embraced jump training as a pivotal part of their fitness regimen, showcasing remarkable progress and achievement.

These stories not only inspire but also provide valuable lessons that can guide beginners on their path toward mastery.

One of the most compelling aspects of jump training success stories is the sheer diversity of backgrounds and goals represented. From athletes seeking to enhance their vertical leap for sports performance to everyday enthusiasts aiming for overall fitness improvement, each journey is unique yet resonant with universal themes of perseverance and growth.

These stories underscore the accessibility of jump training, demonstrating its adaptability to various fitness levels and objectives.

Inspirational stories of jump training success often highlight the tangible results achieved through consistent effort and strategic training. For instance, we encounter individuals who have significantly increased their jump height, surpassed personal records, or achieved specific athletic milestones. These achievements not only showcase the efficacy of structured jump training programs but also serve as tangible markers of progress and success.

Moreover, these narratives delve into the holistic impact of jump training beyond physical prowess. They illuminate how regular jump training can foster resilience, discipline, and mental fortitude, essential qualities that transcend fitness boundaries and manifest in daily life challenges.

By showcasing the multifaceted benefits of jump training, these stories inspire beginners to approach their fitness journey with a holistic mindset, embracing both physical and mental growth.

Real-life applications and transformations captured in jump training success stories provide invaluable insights into the practical implementation of training principles.

These stories often detail the specific exercises, routines, and progression strategies employed by successful jumpers, offering actionable guidance for beginners. Whether it's incorporating plyometric drills, optimizing rest and recovery, or fine-tuning techniques, these narratives serve as practical blueprints for achieving success in jump training.

Furthermore, jump training success stories illuminate the transformative potential of consistent effort and dedication over time. They showcase individuals who have transcended initial challenges, navigated setbacks, and emerged stronger and more resilient.

These stories serve as powerful reminders that progress is a journey marked by perseverance and continuous learning, encouraging beginners to stay committed to their goals despite obstacles.

Lessons learned from experienced jumpers encapsulate invaluable wisdom gained from firsthand experiences and trials. These lessons encompass technical insights into optimizing jump mechanics, practical tips for injury prevention and recovery, as well as mental strategies for overcoming performance barriers. By distilling these lessons into actionable advice, experienced jumpers empower beginners to navigate their training journey with confidence and informed decision-making.

case studies and success stories in jump training for beginners offer a rich tapestry of inspiration, practical wisdom, and transformative narratives.

By immersing in these stories, beginners gain not only motivation but also tangible strategies and insights to embark on their journey towards jump training mastery.

Conclusion

Jumping exercises for beginners are more than just physical movements—they're a gateway to a whole new realm of fitness. Delving into the world of jump training unveils a tapestry of benefits, from enhanced muscular strength and explosive power to improved cardiovascular endurance. But before you take that leap, understanding the nuances is key.

Safety always comes first. Equip yourself with the knowledge of proper form and technique, ensuring each jump is a step towards progress, not injury. Consider the muscles and joints involved, the energy systems at play, and how to gradually increase intensity for optimal results without overtraining.

Designing workouts becomes an art form. Structure sessions smartly, integrating jumps with strength exercises and cardio bursts for a holistic approach. Progression is the name of the game, whether it's vertical leaps, horizontal bounds, or plyometric drills that challenge your explosiveness.

Jump training isn't just about the body; it's a mental game too. Focus, visualize success, and build the mental resilience to push through plateaus. Combine this mental fortitude with proper nutrition and hydration strategies to fuel your performance and aid recovery.

The journey of jump training is marked by milestones—setting goals, overcoming setbacks, and staying motivated through it all. Stories of success from seasoned jumpers inspire and remind us that with dedication and discipline, long-term success is not just a dream but a tangible reality.